THE BUDDING TREE

ASWANI J. NABWENDE

DEDICATION

To women who have suffered conditions that may lead to infertility, still births and miscarriages.

To Men who have stood by these women against all odds.

To my parents Fredrick and Veronicah Aswani for whom family is everything.

ACKNOWLEDGMENTS

Deepest gratitude to God all mighty who enabled me by gifting me with creativity and good health that allowed me to write
THE BUDDING TREE to completion.

Thanks to Benerd Ambani, my Graphic Designer, for his patience towards my demanding nature, for correcting and giving fresh ide-as that birthed the book cover.

To all editors who gave their precious time and untiring efforts to edit and proof read the manuscript, and to beta readers who gave their time to criticize and suggest new ideas for the manuscript.
To you I say thank you.

Is anyone among you suffering? Let him pray.
Is anyone cheerful? Let him sing praise.
Epistle of James –
5:1

*****

My name is Gaudenzia Awiti. You do not know me. Fret not, I am about to introduce myself. My parents gave me four names at birth. I will only tell you about the two that have stuck. These are the names that will usher you into my journey, intro-duce my story and narrate my intricate relationship with death.

I inherited the name Awiti from my father who is a feminist. A rare breed, he allowed his daughters to speak their minds and chase their dreams with little regard to their sexual orientation. It is said that I take after him. I not only look like him but also behave like him. I am like another son to him, so I often sit in his meetings and offer my opinion which is always taken with much value.

My father named me after his grandmother Gaudenzia. He loved to spend most of his time with her as a child. She was not only a great orator but also a fabulous cook.

For all her qualities, my father had no intentions of naming his first child after her until she spotted a pregnant woman in her grandson's hut, and demanded that the child born to be named for her. She had a great third eye.

As fate would have it I took after my great grand-mother, inheriting not only her excellent culinary skills but also her third eye. I had the privilege of knowing my great grandmother. I admired her hard work and self-reliance. She prided herself in being a self-sufficient woman and a proficient barter trader who never lacked something to give.

My great grandmother passed on when I was barely a teenager. Now, I rely on bits of information shared to me by my father and grandfather to better understand a woman whose name I carry on. My grandfather has narrated to me several stories of how my great grandmother survived great pain and anguish. Before holding her first child, she had many miscarriages. She bore each of those loses courageously in her heart at a time when tradition and misguided beliefs overweighed modern medicine.

*****

In African society, some problems are unacceptable as they are taken for curses or witchcraft. This assumption is common among the older generation. The younger generation has been swallowed by advances in modernity, science, and technology. Religious belief has also been of great influence to the youths of today. They live oblivious of the problems in their society that are considered unacceptable. I fall into this category. It took a miscarriage to open my eyes to the strange beliefs around it.

First, I was informed that it was due to my husband's infidelity then it spun to being bewitched by a jealous or evil relative. These beliefs made no sense to us. The gynecologist had explained every-thing. We also knew that most babies were lost in the first trimester and had found our peace.

I spent a lot of time with my mother when I was growing up. To date, she remains my best friend, role model, and number one cheerleader. As her firstborn child, I watched her age like fine wine. My mother taught me to be confident, respectful to self and others and to follow my heart. In this fast-paced world, she ensured that I shared my life with her; from the men I fancied to the ones I committed to. She loved being in control but also allowed me to experience life in full.

I remember vividly an incident that happened when I was nineteen. A boy in my computer class asked me out for an ice-cream date. Unlike my friends, I did not have an official boyfriend yet. It wasn't that I was a shy girl, I was perfectly normal. I just had no interest in boys then. I had no qualms about telling my parents that a boy had asked me out. It did not come as a surprise that my dad did not agree to it, always the protective one, he did not want his little girl to grow up. My mother, on the other hand, was excited. She con-fessed having fears that until that moment, she thought that I would one day join a convent and eventually become a nun. She even gave me money to buy some proper clothes in anticipation for my date. She asked my younger sister, who had an elegant fashion sense to accompany me. I still man-aged to wear my casual jeans, snickers and a jumper for my date. My mother had however ensured that my hair was freshly braided. I looked different. My date bought me ice cream and cake at an ice cream parlor in the city. He was kind enough to buy extra packets for my family. When I got home that evening, my mother and sister were anxiously waiting for me. I spared no detail about my date, opening up about where we went, what we ate, what we talked about and our journey back home.

I had begun a journey that day, a journey of be-coming. Even so, I never thought in my wildest imagination that I would one day sit in my father's living room with my husband, announcing to my parents that they were going to be grandparents. In my parents' world, people married then conceived on their honeymoon. It therefore came as a shock to them when we decided to live together for a year after our marriage ceremony before thinking of starting a family. They did not approve but reluctantly agreed after their pleas fell on deaf ears.

I also did not foresee suffering the same fate as my great grandmother for a second time. I had invited my mother for an ultrasound to surprise her with captured live images and sound waves from my womb, only to be told that I needed to go in for an urgent Dilation and Curettage procedure. Dilation and Curettage, commonly called D&C, is a procedure done to remove a fetus or fetuses from the uterus for one reason or the other.

Medical terms have become easy for me despite the fact that I never attended medical school. I had no interest in human anatomy growing up even though my father tried to push me into it. Eventually, he allowed me to follow my heart. I ended up graduating with a bachelor's degree in media studies. However, I slowly developed an interest in my own anatomy hence doing more research and asking questions about it. Now, I feel I could be a better obstetrician than some physicians I know.

*****

In African society, some problems are unacceptable as they are taken for curses or witchcraft. This assumption is common among the older generation. The younger generation has been swallowed by advances in modernity, science, and technology. Religious belief has also been of great influence to the youths of today. They live oblivious of the problems in their society that are considered unacceptable. I fall into this category. It took a miscarriage to open my eyes to the strange beliefs around it.

First, I was informed that it was due to my husband's infidelity then it spun to being bewitched by a jealous or evil relative. These beliefs made no sense to us. The gynecologist had explained every-thing. We also knew that most babies were lost in the first trimester and had found our peace.

I spent a lot of time with my mother when I was growing up. To date, she remains my best friend, role model, and number one cheerleader. As her firstborn child, I watched her age like fine wine. My mother taught me to be confident, respectful to self and others and to follow my heart. In this fast-paced world, she ensured that I shared my life with her; from the men I fancied to the ones I committed to. She loved being in control but also allowed me to experience life in full.

I remember vividly an incident that happened when I was nineteen. A boy in my computer class asked me out for an ice-cream date. Unlike my friends, I did not have an official boyfriend yet. It wasn't that I was a shy girl, I was perfectly normal. I just had no interest in boys then. I had no qualms about telling my parents that a boy had asked me out. It did not come as a surprise that my dad did not agree to it, always the protective one, he did not want his little girl to grow up. My mother, on the other hand, was excited. She con-fessed having fears that until that moment, she thought that I would one day join a convent and eventually become a nun. She even gave me money to buy some proper clothes in anticipation for my date. She asked my younger sister, who had an elegant fashion sense to accompany me. I still man-aged to wear my casual jeans, snickers and a jumper for my date. My mother had however ensured that my hair was freshly braided. I looked different. My date bought me ice cream and cake at an ice cream parlor in the city. He was kind enough to buy extra packets for my family. When I got home that evening, my mother and sister were anxiously waiting for me. I spared no detail about my date, opening up about where we went, what we ate, what we talked about and our journey back home.

I had begun a journey that day, a journey of be-coming. Even so, I never thought in my wildest imagination that I would one day sit in my father's living room with my husband, announcing to my parents that they were going to be grandparents. In my parents' world, people married then conceived on their honeymoon. It therefore came as a shock to them when we decided to live together for a year after our marriage ceremony before thinking of starting a family. They did not approve but reluctantly agreed after their pleas fell on deaf ears.

I also did not foresee suffering the same fate as my great grandmother for a second time. I had invited my mother for an ultrasound to surprise her with captured live images and sound waves from my womb, only to be told that I needed to go in for an urgent Dilation and Curettage procedure. Dilation and Curettage, commonly called D&C, is a procedure done to remove a fetus or fetuses from the uterus for one reason or the other.

Medical terms have become easy for me despite the fact that I never attended medical school. I had no interest in human anatomy growing up even though my father tried to push me into it. Eventually, he allowed me to follow my heart. I ended up graduating with a bachelor's degree in media studies. However, I slowly developed an interest in my own anatomy hence doing more research and asking questions about it. Now, I feel I could be a better obstetrician than some physicians I know.

*****

Even though we were exhausted during our wed-ding night, my husband and I agreed to attend our evening party for a few minutes. In the midst of loud music and dancing, we knew that it would be easy to slip away into our room. When we went back to our room, we were so tired that we sat in the bathtub, reliving the day and dreaming of the future.

We had spoken about our future before we started planning our marriage. During our premarital counseling sessions, our counselor encouraged us to speak and know each other deeper. He asked us to ponder over a myriad of questions, for instance, would we still love each other if one of us changed physically or if our families became intrusive, or if we did not have children?

At that time, those questions seemed far-fetched. We would never find ourselves in such predicaments, or so we thought. We answered to the affirmative. I must admit that we were well prepared for marriage, the best and the worst of it. Life has however taught me that there is no preparation enough for the realities of what comes after. From differences in ideology to the management of finances, marriage is often set up for failure from the onset. Its success or failure depends entirely on how two individuals raised by different people with different beliefs and lifestyle coexist together. This explains why lasting marriages are viewed as miracles. As we left for our honeymoon, none of these things crossed our mind. We did not anticipate them, so we did not even pray about them.

We were living our best lives, making dreams and working so hard to achieve them that we forgot to count the days after our marriage. For me, nothing much had changed. I was still the same girl. I still loved writing. It was my therapy. In the prior years, I had become a loner which led me to sink into depression hence pushing away important people in my life. My husband had survived the shortlist.

Six months after our nuptials, just when I thought I was settling into the marriage life, I started experiencing irregular menstrual cycles. One particular month, I decided to go for a checkup when my period persisted for more than a fortnight. After consulting my husband I visited a local maternity clinic. In my mind, I thought gynecologists were easily accessible in maternity clinics. I thought it would be a quick fix, all I needed was a few jabs and I would be fine. Instead, I met a young Clinical Officer at the hospital. He inquired whether I had recently traveled among other questions. I wasn't alarmed by the questions because some women experience hormonal imbalances whenever they travel to areas with different weather patterns to what they are used to. I had not traveled in a while, neither had I experienced anything exciting or traumatic enough to alter my cycle. He asked me whether I was trying to conceive, I told him I wasn't. After prescribing some hormonal drugs he assured me that everything would be fine. I was not satisfied.

I had been taking antidepressants but I was sure they were not responsible for my irregular cycles.

I trusted my body. Even though I took the prescription, I had made up my mind to seek a second opinion on the matter. A specialist's opinion is necessary, I thought.

I traveled to see my mum for the weekend after my visit to the clinic. I needed to talk to her about my worries. This trip offered me that chance.

I made many friends in my childhood but my parents were still my confidants. My mum helped me make decisions about my womanhood, relation-ships, family and friends. My dad, on the other hand, helped me make decisions regarding my career, travel destinations and finances. My go-to friend. He always looked after my interests, a fact that caused friction in my household for a long time.

*****

No one tells you that defining the relationship be-tween your father and husband will be difficult. It's even more difficult when you grew up with a strong and supportive father. I was attracted to my husband because of the similarities he shared with my father. He bore the looks that any woman would want including a tall light skinned frame, innocent brown eyes, and a striking smile. His character, beliefs and lifestyle mirrored those of my father. It was as if they had been cut from the same cloth. Sadly, I did not realize this until five years after meeting him. I never took him seriously from the first day at the university. He was the teacher's favorite and had a clique that he hung out with. He sat at the front of the class and had only top per-formers as his close associates. He liked answering questions. It was obvious that he was passionate about school. The only similarity we had is that we were both working and hence struggling to juggle our undergraduate studies with our careers. He had begun drawing close to me, often visiting me at my workplace and constantly reminding me to keep tabs with my studies. Working fulltime had taken a toll on my schooling. He had noticed that I was slacking off.

He was never clear about his intention. Even though he had severally told me that he would marry me someday, I did not take him seriously since that was a decision he had made without consulting me. He therefore remained an acquaintance, just like many other men in the city.

We never lost touch after our graduation, we man-aged to somehow consistently keep in touch with each other and even sneak in a coffee date once in a while. We had grown to have mutual interests so we always had a lot to talk about. Just like my father many years before, he snuck his way into my family by showing up during our family functions and got into my mother's good books. His character secured him a hard-to-cultivate relationship with my father which made him welcomed in our family without fear. Soon after we were married in a sequence of traditional ceremonies that were crowned by a church wedding, a year after our engagement.

Being my father's first daughter to be married, my husband had a tough time negotiating the bride price. Our cultural differences made the already delicate matter a thorn in the flesh. I am often told that I was the first woman in my community whose bride price was negotiated in the midst of women, to date that's a compromise that has not been accepted.

Once, my then fiancé walked out in the middle of negotiations because he could not bear the pressure.

I feel proud when I speak of this matters because, in the end, he proved resolute and finalized the negotiations. I was ready to be his wife. However, he had the patience to wait for a wedding before we started a life together.

*****

After listening to my concerns, my mother advised that I see her doctor; an old man gynecologist and obstetrician who had helped in the delivery of my younger sister two decades ago. At first glance, you would be forgiven for underestimating the grey-haired old man. His tiny eyes and croaky voice made him seem distant, yet he listened keenly and took notes. He asked questions and did proper tests. His meticulous nature has made us friends ever since.

My reproductive system was fine, he assured me. Only for a few tiny cystic sacs that had been observed and which were the cause of the irregular menstrual cycle. At the time I did not understand what it meant.

No explanation made sense to me. I thought I would find solace in Google since it always simplified information for me. Instead, it shook and scared me. I have since learned that Google is neither a good reference point for patients nor for the faint-hearted. While the information provided is relevant, it can be exaggerated and cause utter panic and despair.

Cysts are sacks of unwanted fluids usually found in any part of the body, including the ovary. They are harmless if few but in large numbers when in the ovary they become Polycystic Ovarian Syndrome (PCOS), a hormonal disorder that may delay ovulation and fertility. The cause of PCOS is un-known, though it is common among women with high Body to Mass Index (BMI). Doctors recommend that women keep fit to avoid this condition. I had a few cysts, which were washed away by the tablets I was given. I was back on track, living my best life and waiting for our one year anniversary.

*****

My great grandmother had experienced the same problems years back. Her irregular, prolonged periods made no sense then. Even the facts about her miscarriages may have been misrepresented be-cause the science of medicine was not as developed as it is now. Her first son, my grandfather, who had been sharing this information with me, may not have had the facts correctly because in those days such matters were not discussed by men, especially not the direct offspring of the affected.

My grandfather's sister, who liked me from birth had mentioned her own undocumented problems to me. She speaks fondly about her mother, my great grandmother.

A famous herbalist had been visiting my great grandmother. She made her chew herbal leaves and change her diet, helping her to nurture her pregnancy when she conceived and clean her womb after she had a miscarriage.

My great grandmother was a religious woman, yet another thing we have in common. She kept to herself, apart from the many times she walked into my grandfather's compound to check on her daughter-in-law. Meals were taken seriously, especially when I visited her. She was determined that I go back to the city heavier than I had come.

My great grandmother spoke little about the pains she had to endure, maybe it was because in her eyes I was just a little girl or maybe in those days the problem that women faced was a burden they had to bear silently.

Had I known that I would suffer from the same problems, I would have grown up a bit faster so that I could pick her mind on a few things. How had she survived such pain to raise six children? How did she find the strength to exist in a judgmental society? How did she forget the pain of her previous miscarriage and found the courage to carry another without the surety of whether it would survive or whether she would survive? These questions did not cross my mind when my husband and I decided that it was time to expand our own family. It never occurred to me that they would ever cross my mind.

By this time, there was no trace of cysts in my reproductive system. My conception had long been approved by my doctor.

The conception was easy since my menstrual cycle had gone back to normal. It was thus easy to know my fertility window. The women at my local Anglican church played a big role in this by getting me a book on sexuality, family and family planning methods.

A month later when I took that long-awaited pregnancy test it turned positive. I was over-whelmed by emotions at what I knew from the beginning was a miracle. In the washroom where I was, tears of joy were streaming down my face. My breathing increased and the smile on my face widened as I looked at that tiny Human

Chorionic Gonadotropin (HCG) strip. My hands tenderly held on my tummy, not sure where to specifically place them so that my baby would feel my presence. My husband was busy in the living room. I knew he would be excited to hear the news, but I wanted to make it special by surprising him. I like making mountains out of ant hills. This was after all more than a mere ant hill so a mountain kind of attention was necessary.

In the living room, my husband's eyes were fixated on the television but I knew that his mind was probably wondering why we had argued a few minutes ago. Before I went into the washroom, we had argued about something that I couldn't quite recall. On our first year of marriage, we had our own fair share of petty arguments just as our counselor had anticipated. I loved my toothpaste pressed from the bottom, he didn't care, as long as teeth got cleaned. I am very conscious of where I place things. He calls it Obsessive Compulsive Disorder (OCD), I call it neatness. He loved his food without spices, I loved mine marinated, garnished and spice filled. So, our petty differences had us not talking at that memorable moment of our lives.

I walked out of the washroom smiling, still plotting how I would break the news to him. He must have wondered what had happened in the washroom that suddenly lifted my moods. I tried to tease him out of his foul mood, but he was having none of it. If only he knew what I wanted to tell him.

It took me a month and a half to reveal my little secret to my husband. Procrastination became a game. My husband loved me truly and deeply. Like the African man he was, he felt it was in his place to provide for his family, in this case, to provide for me. Despite growing up in different environments, him in the village and I in the city, he easily adjusted to my lifestyle. He supported my decisions concerning our family. I had a big say on the type of furniture we had, the area we resided, the people we associated with as well as the design of our future home.

I had visited his house many times before our marriage. I knew that after we got married, I would change everything in it. The furniture was old fashioned, not to be confused with the antique kind. His dining table was leaning precariously on one side of the wall in the living room of his one bed-roomed house. There was a gas cylinder beneath it and a cooking burner on top of it. The only three cooking pans in the house were neatly arranged beside the sink in the kitchen. A typical bachelor's pad. I wanted to make a home out of it, to bring my contemporary bohemian style and make it a place where we could raise our children.

Our first fight was as a result of me moving his items without his permission. We were caught be-tween what I wanted versus what he thought was proper. I argued that I was in order, as a woman, to make the home. He objected saying that since he was the head of the home he should have a major say on things that happened there.

Such arguments would leave us not talking for days hence the reason why I found it easy to procrastinate sharing the good news with him. I knew that my secret would not last very long. Pregnancy is a secret that speaks for itself, it was just a matter of time.

I casually invited my husband for our first antenatal clinic, then broke the news a few minutes be-fore we saw the doctor. His reaction was not immediate so I could not read his mind. He neither looked surprised nor excited about the news. I watched as his thoughts wandered to a place far away from where we were.

Women and men process information differently. For me, this was a natural step, something we had planned, anticipated and prepared for. Already I was secretly writing little notes for my unborn child, explaining what he meant to me and his father and how we have great dreams for him. I explained to him how I could not wait to hold him in my arms. Any time I passed by the mirror I stopped to see how many inches my belly had grown. Months later, I imagined that I would be stopping by the same mirror with my child, admiring the two of us. I couldn't wait for his first mile-stones.

The news of an additional member of the family meant something else to my husband. It meant in less than nine months, he had to put everything in order so as to give us the best life. He did not have a car yet. How were we to move around with an infant? How would he provide for his growing family? He had thoughts of building a home before his firstborn arrived. Anxiety started to build up. Would he pull all these feats in nine months?

Even though he did not have to do all those things, he still felt pressured. On the other hand, I did not feel the rush. I just knew that our lives would never be the same.

Our gynecologist was happy about the news of our pregnancy. He immediately ordered an ultrasound.

Everything looked okay except for a few cysts that were not life-threatening. Once implantation has happened, cysts hardly interfere with a pregnancy. In fact, a specific kind of cyst is welcome in pregnancy as it helps in sustaining the embryo. My doctor, however, recommended that I take some medication to dissolve the cysts. He also pre-scribed antenatal drugs, which included some vitamins and folic acid.

The sonographer reported that I was just five weeks pregnant, even though I believed I was closing in on my second trimester. The confusion in timelines between the sonographer and the pregnant woman is taken seriously in the medical world. There has been unquestionable evidence that a woman knows her body best and if she insists on something, there is a high probability that she is right. For this reason, we were booked in for another ultrasound three weeks later. By that time, it was expected that the embryo would be grown enough to not only give us an Anticipated Date of Delivery (ADD) but also have a strong heartbeat. We were hopeful and happy. By the time we were leaving the clinic, even my husband was beginning to accept the idea of fatherhood.

*****

My husband lost his father two years before our marriage. His mother had passed on while he was still a teenager. My pregnancy was a big blessing for him. He felt that this was a chance for him to not only name our child after one of his parents but also to continue their lineage.

Since his father's death, my husband has had to make decisions on his own, some of which he failed at and others he prided in, like his young family. Although he missed his parents, he felt he had a second chance when he met mine and they created a bond similar to that of a child and his biological parents.

We, therefore, made a deliberate decision to have dinner with our parents at least once a month. We used that time to catch up on our lives and ex-changed notes. Our parents were no longer just parents but friends and role models. They had been married for more than three decades, survived the test of time and overcome the challenges of inter-tribal marriages. We sought their counsel, celebrated our achievements with them and asked for their guidance during tough times.

We had decided to break the good news to them that they were going to be grandparents during our next visit. Since I was their child, my husband decided it would be awkward for him to break the news especially in the presence of his father-in-law. The onus was on me to break the news. Despite always being open with my parents, this was still a daunting task.

I needed to be tactical, I needed to have a plan. These are, after all, African parents and as modern as they may be, you cannot predict their reaction on receiving the news in our presence.

I bought a wonderful key holder for my mother and inscribed the following sentence on it, 'Dear grandmother, please pray for me that I may get here safely early next year'. In it was watermarked photo of my husband and I. As for my father, I just needed to tell him. Like my husband, he was too old fashioned to understand the news any other way. I decided I would show him our doctor's report. It would be easier for him to figure it out since he was a medical practitioner.

I couldn't help thinking what it would have been like if my great grandmother was alive to witness this. How happy would she have been to see 'her-self' get pregnant again? I am sure I would have been placed on a strict diet. I won't even mention how furious her prayers for me and my unborn child would have been.

My mum was in the kitchen preparing chapati when we walked into the house. She loved to feed my husband, and my husband loved my mother's chapati so much that each time we visited we had to carry some to our house.

I joined my mother in the kitchen while my husband, my father, and my brothers indulged in a tet a tet in the living room. We enjoyed a wonderful meal together and after that, I announced that I had important news to share. Suddenly, I had everyone's attention.

I walked to my father and handed him an envelope that contained our medical report, then handed the key holder to my mother. What followed was a silence so stealth that we could hear each other breathe. We watched our parents keenly for any reaction. My father was the first to raise his head. He looked at his wife and nodded slightly. My mother soon followed. She looked at me and gave me a mild smile. We all felt awkward.

"Dad, have you read what the doctor wrote?" I probed.

He did not answer. Instead, he sighed. I know my father well. In fact, I prided in being able to read his mind. As I looked into his blank face, I could tell he was happy. In his heart, he was probably dancing to La Macarena by the famous Los Del Rio and struggling to keep his face straight. As for my mother, it was only a matter of time before she gave away her emotions. Like me, she was not good at hiding her feelings. She was probably waiting for my father to react before she could.

This day reminded my husband of the day he came home to officially ask my father for my hand in marriage. He could not read what the old man was thinking as he sat there with him waiting for his word. That day my husband wished the earth would swallow him whole. The silence was deafening. Were it not for his cousin and best friend, he would have bolted out of our house, never to come back.

Like that day, my father was happy, even though his expression said otherwise.

During my pregnancy, I carried myself with much caution. I sat strategically inside the matatu when-ever I was traveling. If I was asked to move to accommodate an extra person on my seat, I alighted and waited for another vehicle or called for a taxi. At work, I added a pillow on my chair to give my back more support. I also wore loose clothes.

I spent my spare time shopping for baby clothes and learning more about the gestation period.

Although I did not have any cravings, I loathed anything that had cheese or onions. Their smell repulsed me. I began to avoid colleagues who carried their lunch to work and often I chewed on oranges to prevent feeling nauseous.

The three weeks before our next appointment seemed like an eternity. My mind was glued to the tiny human growing in my belly. Not a single day did I forget he was there nor stop praying and writing to him. One day when my unborn baby was grown up, I would reveal all these letters to him for him to read and know exactly how I felt about him. I wanted him to know that he was wanted and loved even before his arrival. My letters to him were as raw and open as I felt. I wanted him to know me in such a deep manner.

*****

There are many beliefs used to predict the gender of an unborn child. Even before the ultrasound was invented, midwives predicted the sex of a child from the way the mother behaved at the be-ginning of her pregnancy. Morning sickness, cravings, stress levels and how high or low a mother carried the baby were some of the traditional methods used to determine the sex of an unborn child.

I once broke the news of my pregnancy to a friend who insisted that I was carrying a boy since my stomach was hanging low. If it was a girl, my stomach would be higher than it was. I did not believe her because it was still too early to tell the gender of my unborn child.

Besides, I have always had a potbelly which hangs low from my stomach and which can be confused for pregnancy.

My father, even though he didn't speak about my pregnancy, had previously pointed out the recur-rent happenings in our family. All my paternal uncles and aunties had girls as their firstborn children. My family therefore expected that I would have a girl. On the other hand, all of my husband's sib-lings had boys as their firstborn children. They too expected that I would have a boy.

Despite all this my motherly instinct had me convicted that I was carrying a boy. So much so that it would have been a great disappointment if I went for the ultrasound and discovered that I was carrying a girl.

*****

I had already joined various social media groups for expectant mothers. Thanks to technology, I had found a group of women whom our delivery would be at almost similar times. We would walk the journey of pregnancy together. A childhood friend, whom we got married at the same time was also expectant. We constantly exchanged notes and updated each other on our life-changing experiences.

She was yet to start on her antenatal visits, yet here I was getting ready for my second appointment. I read the many experiences that women wrote concerning their pregnancies on these social groups. Some were having a smooth ride while some experienced harrowing morning sicknesses. Others were on bed rest while others had miscarried.

I felt sorry for the women who had miscarried. It must have been tough, I thought. However, I also commended their courage to share their experience with strangers on social media. It was telling to note their advice on the red flags that women needed to look out for during their pregnancy.

Until this point, nothing about my great grand-mother came to mind. She was long gone, except for a picture of her that was hung on the wall in my grandfather's house. In my father's house, there was another picture of her, seated on a chair, with a kettle of tea on the table. She loved tea.

As I thought about the women who had lost their pregnancies, a thought crossed my mind. What if it happened to me? What if I lost this baby that was already the center of my universe? I quickly brushed the thought away. How dare I harbor such thoughts? I immediately rebuked them, said my prayers and went to bed.

I am a night owl, but once I hit the bed, I sleep like a baby. I loved my sleep so much that I be-came cranky to anyone who dared interrupt.

This particular night, I could not sleep. Several times my sleep was interrupted by nightmares. Finally, I woke up. Eyes wide open I lay in bed facing the ceiling. I could not vividly remember my nightmares so I allowed my mind to wander as I waited for sleep to sweep me away once again. That did not happen.

I began imagining how the life of motherhood would be. Still, I felt a niggling feeling that some-thing was not right. I felt like a tree that had its fruit forcefully plucked off of it.

My husband who was by my side was sleeping soundly, snoring away in a rhythmic manner. He was a heavy sleeper. Often, I joked that someone could carry him in his sleep for miles without him waking up. He must be in dreamland by now, I thought. I was now fully awake.

Since sleep was not forthcoming, I needed to pass time. I decided to empty my bladder. I wasn't necessarily pressed, I just needed to get out of bed and do something. Slowly I rose from the bed, keen not to switch on the lights in our bedroom so as not to interrupt my husband's sleep. I walked into the washroom, switched on the lights and pulled down my pajamas. Before I could do anything, a strange object fell from between my legs. Was I still asleep? I pinched myself to ensure I was not dreaming.

Quickly, I rose from the toilet seat to see what had fallen into the bowl. A clear tennis sized clump of tissue was floating in the clear toilet water. Curios as to what it might be, I wore a glove and re-moved the mass from the toilet. I wasn't in any pain so I couldn't possibly have had a miscarriage, my mind raced. I had heard stories of strange happenings in pregnancy, but nothing was close to this. Was it my baby's amniotic sack? I asked myself. Questions filled my mind. I decided to go back to bed and wait for the break of dawn since I was not in pain. I would visit the hospital for quick consultation in the morning. I did not panic; panic was not good for pregnancy. I needed to stay calm. I woke my husband up gently and informed him of the strange happening. As we went back to sleep, I felt a strong urge to ask my husband to pray for us. I believed only God understood the secret happenings inside a woman's body. Therefore only He could be relied on to watch over me. My husband obliged, uttering a solemn prayer before we went back to sleep.

*****

I have heard many stories about the pain women in labor go through. My best friend has two sons. I have watched them grow from birth. The morning after her first delivery, she narrated to me how much pain she felt pushing her son out of her body. The pain was too much to bear that she subconsciously plucked a handful of her hair off her head. This must be what is called a labor of love.

The pain that a woman experiences at childbirth have often been likened to twenty bones being fractured at a go. Yet women still have the strength to get second, third and even fourth babies. Amazingly, despite all their pain, wailing, shouting and even stripping, women hardly shed a tear during labor. Tears were forbidden in the de-livery room because it was believed that tears welcomed death into the room that was meant to facilitate an incoming new life.

A sharp pain woke me just as I was beginning to doze off. At first, it was a bearable cramp, almost similar to a menstrual period cramp. A few seconds later it worsened.

I had never been in labor before but this sure felt like 20 bones being fractured. I felt as if my back was detaching itself from the rest of my body. My pulse was becoming weaker. I could feel my joints lose their strength. The pain was so much that I could not raise my voice to awaken my already sleeping husband. I knew something had terribly gone wrong. Tears freely rolled down my cheeks as I struggled to stretch my hand and wake my husband up.

My mind could not process what was happening. Had we not left God in charge when we went to sleep? Might the prayers have fallen on deaf ears? Had I smothered my pregnancy so much that it found me undeserving? Was I overthinking? May-be I was just having a reaction to something. Tears kept falling down my chubby cheeks uncontrollably. I finally managed to wake my husband up. One look at me was enough for him to jump into action. Quickly, he pulled a jacket that was lying on the floor and left the room to call a taxi. I rolled myself off the bed. The pain was too much to bear, so on my fours, I followed my husband into the living room, begging him to hurry. I was holding onto the hope that if we could get to the hospital on time, our unborn child would be saved.

I looked back and noticed a trail of blood all the way from the bedroom. My heart broke. How had God allowed this to happen? Had He forgotten me? Was I undeserving of His grace? Had I done something wrong? It took us five minutes to leave the house. I lay on the back seat of a Nissan Bluebird car as my husband took the co-driver's seat. He did not say a word to the driver. The driver sped off. He knew that he needed to be at the hospital as soon as possible.

By the time the driver stopped at the entrance of the hospital, the pain in my body could not com-pare to that in my heart, soul and mind. As he and my husband pulled me out of the vehicle onto a stretcher that a nurse was holding, I could no longer hold my pain.

I was neither in control of my body nor my mind. Using the little strength that I had left, I let out a wail. I was wheeled straight into the emergency room as my husband filled the administration de-tails. The doctor on call and my husband joined me in the emergency room just as the sonographer was winding up. She looked straight into my eyes and whispered, "I am sorry."

"We need to get you into the theater", the doctor said as the sonographer stepped aside.

I could not listen or watch as the doctor pointed on the ultrasound screen and explained to my husband that there were tissues in my womb that needed to be removed through an evacuation procedure.

I was certain that God had not only left my body but also my household.

Maybe if I had stopped my tears from flowing, I would have saved my child, I thought.

I blacked out and woke up at midday in a maternity ward. The evacuation procedure had already been done. The doctor explained that the procedure entailed sucking the tissues from the womb using a manual vacuum aspirator.

It was a painful and intrusive procedure. I am grateful that I had been on anesthesia. Previously, women like my great grandmother would have been tied on a hospital bed with their legs wide open as a medical practitioner inserted her hand through the vagina and scraped off all the remains of a pregnancy.

I couldn't imagine the pain these women endured during this procedure. My great grandmother had endured too many of such that she lost count. Shockingly, she still managed to bring forth six babies.

*****

The night before, I had been having dreams and plans for my unborn. Now, all that was left was a memory. As I lay in bed facing the roof in my blue hospital outfit, many thoughts raced through my mind. My eyes were still pouring out the feelings in my heart. I hardly noticed the other four women in the ward.

"She is so beautiful," the woman lying on the bed next to mine said.

"Who?" I asked amidst tears.

"I just had a baby girl," she continued, "She's the copyright image of her father."

"Congratulations! We thank God for safe delivery," I responded.

"I actually had a cesarean section, my baby was in a breech position."

Lucky her, I thought. I would have taken a baby in breech position over a dead one any day.

"I cannot wait for us to visit the nursery. Did you have a boy or a girl?" she asked oblivious of the wounds she was opening.

I felt as if a knife had been stabbed through my chest and twisted infinitely. I did not answer. My silence made her whisper her apologies. I smiled and maintained my mum. She understood and did not probe further. I shivered at the thought of having to answer this question over and over again.

My mother was the first to visit. She shared my pain, joining me in my tears. We hugged and held onto each other for a while before I let go and slumped on my bed. I was still groggy from the fading anesthesia. I neither wanted to talk nor be around anyone. All I wanted to do was wallow in my own pain, stay in bed and somehow regain my pregnancy.

I could not go back home knowing well that the ball of tissue was still in my washroom. How could I flash it down the toilet knowing fully well what it was? How could I even look at it?

All this time, my husband stayed quiet. He must have been struggling with his own grief, unsure of what to say to me. He did not come near me, his brother did. He kept his distance. He processed my discharge and brought me a fresh change of clothes. We were heading home to start our lives again, just the two of us.

*****

My great grandmother would have had an evacuation procedure and as soon she left hospital gone straight to the farm to tend to her crops. She would have carried water on her head and hidden her innermost feelings to herself, never to bring them up again. If she were here, she would have accused me of eating too much fast food and using the washing machine too much. She would have blamed all my recovery struggles to modern lifestyle.

I knew I would be on a diet of porridge and oxtail soup if she was here.

I was conscious of what I was supposed to do. The doctor had advised me to avoid heavy duties so as to allow my body to recover. He explained to me that I would experience bleeding for a while before my menstrual cycle returned to its normalcy. Despite my mid and lower back being weaker and painful, my body was prepared for recovery.

Two days later, I reported back to work, ready to occupy my mind and bury my hurt feelings, just like my great grandmother had done years before me. My husband had called in at work and explained my absence to my superior. However five minutes after settling in, I was summoned into the administration office and fired for absconding du-ty. I was being released from the one place I thought would destruct me from my pain. I wanted to put up a legal fight, but I did not have the courage to relive what had happened to me.

I packed my belongings, bid my colleagues' good-bye, called my husband and left the premises. I now had time in my hands, enough to be haunted by my thoughts; enough to go through every one of my actions and try to determine which one could have cost me my pregnancy.

I spent most of my time crying in the washroom.

Severally my husband caught me huddled in a corner of our house sobbing. I intentionally avoided anyone who would feel sorry for me. I knew most meant well but the word sorry cut through me like a knife on butter. After a miscarriage, a woman's hormones are usually heightened, which causes mixed feelings and emotions. Grief is inevitable.

I decided to visit my doctor who was surprised by the new development. He had not learned of my miscarriage yet. It's easy to assume, that after years and years of attending to patients and seeing too many sick-nesses, miscarriages and deaths, a doctor would not be moved when something bad happens to his patient. My doctor was shocked at my misfortune.

"I am sorry," he said after I explained to him the ordeal I went through. I wanted to find out more about what happened to me. Him being my gynecologist, he would know more.

"Doctor, what really happened to me?" I asked as I settled down in his consultation room.

I needed him to justify the loss, to tell me what I did wrong or what he missed on my first appointment. "It's not your fault. Do not blame yourself," he said as if he was reading my mind.

"It's quite common for infants to die during the first trimester." he continued, "There is absolutely nothing you would have done to prevent it."

"But I wasn't on the first trimester," I insisted.

The difference in the age of my pregnancy be-tween me and my sonographer had not been re-solved yet.

According to the measurements of the fetus during our first antenatal clinic, it was determined that I was just five weeks pregnant while according to my last menstrual period I believed I was nine weeks pregnant.

"Then it must be a blighted ovum," he exclaimed in a light bulb moment.

A blighted ovum is a condition where the amniotic sac and the placenta grow but the baby doesn't. That, he explained would be a logical reason as to why the sonographer and I reported different ages for the pregnancy. There was no justifiable reason as to why a miscarriage could occur in the first trimester. The Doctor advised that I continue taking the antenatal drugs to assist my body in healing. After a few examinations, he assured me that I would be okay to carry another pregnancy to term.

I went home and continued taking the drugs that I had been given; drugs that I had initially taken with much pride but which were now a constant reminder that I was not going to be a parent in nine months anymore.

I was twenty-seven years old when I had a miscarriage. Medically, I was still young and fertile enough to deliver as many children as I wanted. The doctors often advise women to have children earlier in life because fertility decreases with age and the risk of pregnancy complications is low. My mother had her children early. By the time she was my age, she already had four children. After that flurry, she did not have more children. We all were born at intervals of two years, so we were all toddlers at the same time. My mother consequently struggled to run errands with all of us demanding her attention. Out of concern, strangers had ad-vised my mother to consider family planning methods. My mother's body recovered slowly from the rigours of giving birth such that by the time she was 29 you'd mistake her for a teenager. She has always looked younger than her age. Better yet, she raised her children together.

My mother does not clearly understand the kind of troubles I faced. She likes to blame everything on our modern lifestyle, just like my great grandmother would.

She did not experience any troubles with her pregnancies. Her four children were born through normal delivery, eighty fractured bones in total.

After I got married, my plan was to have my four children before I got to my mid-thirties. I had hoped to have a life like that of my mother. In that life, miscarriages did not exist.

The doctor had informed me that in three months I could try having another child if I wanted. A woman who has undergone an evacuation procedure has a higher chance of conceiving than a normal woman. So, all indications showed that I could get pregnant soon if I chose to.

*****

The election period in my country always strikes fear and terror in the hearts of people. Past elections had caused havoc, loss of property and lives further dividing us along our feeble tribal lines. Many families had to move from their homes and start over because their property had been vandalized or stolen and lives put at risk. It was no surprise that every time elections drew close, families moved back to their rural homes so as to be near their people. No one was taking risks.

Elections came just two weeks after I miscarried. We were caught between a rock and a hard place. Do we travel upcountry or stay put? To further complicate matters, my father had asked us to be home during that period to reduce worry and dis-tress. As his children, we were expected to oblige. We, however, were aware that I was to avoid traveling for long distances so as allow my womb and back to heal.

The lining of my womb had been scraped off in the process of evacuation hence any bouncing, friction or strain would have prolonged the healing process. This would consequently cause strain to the back. I opted to take the twelve-hour journey anyway. Normally, I would have traveled during the night, do my business during the day, assess the situation and leave for the city following night. This time, I chose to stay in the village a little longer with the hope that the fresh air, fresh pro-duce and serenity would accelerate my recovery.

We also thought that it was important to give each other some space. I felt abandoned by my husband during my grieving period. He did not like seeing me cry and he voiced his feelings. He felt that I was exaggerating my emotions. He also struggled to understand why I did not want people to come over to our house and visit.

Men and women grieve differently. For me, every time I felt choked up by my feelings, I wailed and tore until I felt better. During this period, all I wanted was to be held by my husband and be assured that everything would be okay.

As for my husband, he grieved differently. For him, I came first. So, he had to put away his sorrows to take care of mine. He had to stay strong because he did not want to make me feel sadder than I already was. I did not understand that. I wanted him to be open, vulnerable and true to his emotions, just like I was.

While at the village, I spent most of my time in the shade of an old mango tree. I remember restlessly sitting under the same tree with my great grand-mother when I was just a child. She tried to make me sit still but I wanted to run around and play with my cousins.

Under this same tree, my grandfather had told me stories of his parents, his mother especially. Where I come from, reincarnation is viewed as a possible occurrence. Severally I have been told that I share the same characters as my great grandmother. Were it not for the fact that we met and lived in a shared timeline, I would have been accused of being her reincarnate.

Under this tree, I remember being told stories of how my great grandmother suffered in her quest to have a child; how she had had several miscarriages and stillbirths. I remember the stories of the doc-tor who assisted my great grandmother through what is now called an evacuation procedure. Then, words like evacuation and antenatal care were just jargons.

That doctor's name was Awiti. She was a famous herbalist who would perhaps have been a renowned gynecologist and obstetrician to-day. Awiti only had one condition; that one of the many babies she helped bring forth be named after her. The sex of the baby did not matter.

When my grandfather was born, he was named Awiti. Consequently, his children took up the same name and passed it on to their children. I bear such a name, directly from my father, but indirectly from the suffering of my great grandmother.

*****

My husband and I spent our second marriage anniversary apart. I in the village and him in the city. At this point celebrating marriage was not a priori-ty to us. It had not brought any good tidings to us, especially in the ending year. Although we did not blame each other for our loss, we did not clear each other of the same blame either. We had a strain so strong that I began thinking of many other people who would have made better partners.

On the list were some of my close friends who I had known for a long time, longer than I had known my husband. I grew up a conservative girl, but I had a knack of attracting the right kind of friends in my circles.

During my school years, I happened to be among the few girls who performed well in school. In those days we sat according to our performance in the classroom. I only associated myself with the people I sat with, the majority of those were boys. I grew close to some of those boys over time to an extent that I thought I would end up marrying one of them. Those were the ones crossing my mind now. I imagined they would be more considerate to my feelings than my husband, after all, they knew me better. I regretted not having tolerated the idea when I was still single.

When in pain, a lot of crazy things come to your mind. They call it Post Traumatic Stress Disorder (PTSD). The emotions, without logic, decide who is good and who is bad.

I know this for sure. Before I got married, I went into depression. It was a difficult time that cost me a few years of my youths. During that period, I neither wanted to be around my friends or family. I intentionally misplaced my phone so as not to be reached. I avoided them like a plague. I felt like the universe owed me something better, the same feeling I was having when I decided that my husband was not worth enough of a partner.

On my return to our home, I discovered that there was more to fix than I imagined. A month quickly passed without me feeling better. My husband tried his best. He was saying all the right words. He tried his best to let me know that I was loved and cared for. Any normal person would realize that many men knew not how to handle pain as he had. He was strong, not just for himself, but for me too. He was patient and tolerant with me as I healed.

However, healing is one thing while forgetting is another.

"Don't let it go too far, don't lose us like we lost our young one," my husband said one evening. "In fact, let's have another baby," he added.

There is no single day that I have forgotten of my first pregnancy. I often imagine how life would have been had my son survived my hostile womb. This has never stopped me from celebrating other mothers. I never sulk during children's celebrations or burst into tears. I find enough grace to join in their celebration and share their happiness.

We still held onto our dreams. Mine was to have my children while still young while my husband' was that one year after our marriage we would go on a childbearing marathon. We waited for another two months to pass, and we were pregnant again. There was no excitement in announcing this news to my partner. I did not have the formula to do it and I did not want to wait. I simply told him the first chance I got. It was confusing, we did not know whether we were happy, worried or sad. How were we to celebrate this pregnancy when we had just lost another? How could we forget? We doubted everything we did. I chose not to work for a while so as to give my pregnancy enough attention.

This time, we neither wrote any letters to our un-born nor spoke about it, just in case a bad spell was still hovering around. We also did not tell any-one about the news apart from our gynecologist. Tests were done with much keenness. There were no cysts, nothing that would indicate any risk for the baby. Even with a clear medical record, we still worried and reported to the hospital whenever any issues arose, however minor. We were determined to have this child, by whatever means.

*****

I thought carefully about informing my sister about my second pregnancy. Even though she was younger than me, she always had been a great part of my life and bore my burdens with enormous grace. After the miscarriage, my sister had sacrificed her time to stay with me and take care of the things that I couldn't at the time. Like my mother, my sister bore my grief as if it were her own. We not only shared our grief but also interests and friends. We have looked out for each other since we knew of each other. Informing my sister of my pregnancy also meant that I was passing on the same worry I had to her. My sister is a young woman, single and she enjoys dating and discovering herself. I always prayed and hoped that my experiences would not scare her off living and enjoying her life.

While it was important that women support each other through difficult times, it was also important that they enjoy their good times. It would be selfish of me to inform her of things that may scare her of marriage. I decided that I would not tell her about my pregnancy, not to deprive her of the joy but to spare her from the worries.

My own misfortune had made me protective of my female friends and relatives. I wanted them to use my experiences and visit gynecologists for check-ups and preventive healthcare. Apart from PCOS and

Endometriosis, Cervical cancer has become the other great risk to women. I would wish for my sister to be exposed to such information. Prevention is, after all, better than cure

For most women, the first antenatal visit is usually when the pregnancy is between 8 weeks to 12 weeks. But for a woman who carries a potential rainbow baby, it is advised that she reports to the hospital as soon as she finds out she is expectant. This is to ensure that any preventive measure is taken and all tests are done in time in an effort to keep the pregnancy.

The risk of a miscarriage is high when a pregnancy is below 14 weeks. The chances reduce to less than one percent as the pregnancy progresses. Women who have suffered one miscarriage have a 20 per-cent chance of having another miscarriage. That chance increases to 28 percent after the second miscarriage. After the third miscarriage, the chances of a miscarriage increase to 48 percent and so on.

This explains why my great grandmother suffered so many miscarriages. I could not imagine bearing that kind of pain, and even though I was worried about my second pregnancy, I held on to hope and believe that God would make it successful.

There are days I wished I would forget that I was pregnant. Those days were few, but when they came, they gave me so much relief. It would be safer if I didn't know, I felt that would give my child a fighting chance.

*****

On one of my hospital visits, we noticed that my weight was more than expected. I was worried, but the doctor informed me that it was okay. There was nothing we could have done anyway. Expectant women are not allowed to lose weight, let alone try to. We felt comforted when a nurse in-formed us that there could be an explanation for the unexpected weight gain. The possibility of a dual pregnancy. The idea of having twins was welcomed. It signaled a double blessing. Even though we knew that the woman's genes are the determinants of whether or not a couple could have twins, we had entertained the possibility because my husband was a twin. He and his fraternal brother have shared with me many stories of their childhood. Stories of their struggles for attention, their fights and their struggles building their individual personalities. Stories of their parents and how they contributed to the adults that they are today. Stories that I find funny and which I would have wanted my own children to live through.

The idea excited us. We could not wait for the pregnancy to grow so that we may ascertain if that was the reason for my unexpected weight gain. Even before our marriage, we were excited at the idea of expanding our family. Many times, we reflected on the kind of parents we wanted to be-come and the names we would give our children.

One day as I dozed off in the living room, I had an exciting dream. I was carrying a round-faced bubbly light-skinned baby girl while taking a stroll with my eldest brother. We were laughing and making jokes. We seemed happy. I held her up, smiled and passed her on to my brother to carry. We then continued to walk, the child content in his arms. The dream was brief, but it never left my mind. I was less than a year married and my broth-er was just winding up his studies.

Myth has it that if you want a dream to come true you keep it to yourself. If you want it to fade away you tell it to others. I do not believe in myths. The joy of having that dream could not allow me to keep it to myself. I informed my mother and my sister while hanging out with them. I told them something good was about to happen. I would first have it, but my brother would keep it. I assured them that it was something good because there was a child involved. Something in my heart gave me the conviction that children in dreams were a good thing. This was way back in the formative years of my marriage. By the time I was carrying my second pregnancy, I was well into my fourth year of marriage. My brother had long graduated and was settled back at home so much that he was planning to marry his long-term girlfriend.

No one except for our doctor knew about our second pregnancy. We were keen not to count our chicks before they hatched. We had already been to two antenatal appointments, the third one would be at 10 weeks.

I dreaded going to the toilet however unavoidable it was. Each time I went in there, I was afraid I would spot blood. Bleeding is not good for pregnancy, except for implantation bleeding which happens very early in the pregnancy for some women. Any form of bleeding or discharge is considered dangerous. For this reason, I was quite alarmed to see a pink discharge when I visited the toilet one day. We immediately rushed to the hospital. After tests were done, I was given some drugs and sent home. I was also instructed to stay in bed and avoid heavy duties. I obliged. The rea-son for the discharge was unknown, but the doc-tor assured me that if I followed his instructions I would be fine.

I stayed in bed, my husband taking over the majority of the house chores. I took this as the most sacrificial act of love. Majority of African men do not enjoy house chores.

While they love to eat, they would rather be served than go to the kitchen. They hate dirty dishes. I felt really blessed to have a husband who would take care of the kitchen duties while I stayed in bed and rested. Even though the discharge did not stop, we still followed the doctor's order. On the tenth week, we reported to the hospital as advised. It was our next appointment. The plan was for my husband and me to go for the checkup, then meet up with our mother to inform her of the new developments. We decided to take an ultrasound before we saw our doctor. It was a routine procedure. Even after we saw the doctor, he would still have sent us for the ultrasound before he could decide on any diagnosis. It would be wise for us to take our ultra-sound results with us to his office.

My mother was already on her way to meet us. My husband had to rush for a meeting after the appointment. Since he was already running late, I allowed him to go as I stayed in line to wait for the test. I took plenty of water in preparation. A full bladder usually allows for better images during the ultrasound. If my bladder was not filled it would have resulted in a Trans-Vaginal Ultrasound, an-other of medicines most intrusive tests. I did not want that, so I took my water without limitations.

The continuous discharge that I had been experiencing made me nervous. I did not know whether to expect bad news or good news. Thankfully, my mother arrived just as I was about to go in. She stood on one corner of the room as the sonographer put a cold jelly on my stomach. He then placed the machine on my belly and on the monitor, we began to observe.

I could not hear any heartbeat, and neither could I see any movement on the monitor. I did not say a word, I just lay there silently and hoped that I did not have enough experience to know how the ma-chine worked. Usually, the sonographer explains everything as soon as he sees it on the monitor. This time he took time to respond. That too, I ignored, hoping that my uterus was so complicated that he had to take more time to interpret what he was seeing.

"See this?" he finally broke the silence pointing at the monitor. "This is the fetus. Do you see where it is? This is where it is meant to be," he continued while still pointing to the monitor. "It has already detached itself from the umbilical cord and is on its way out. I am deeply sorry." He landed the blow.

I could not believe it. I stayed glued at the monitor for a while. My mother must have moved closer as I was zoned out and held my hand as the sonographer left to print and prepare the results. I did not hear him when he emphasized how urgent we should see the doctor. I finally arose from the examination bed, straightened my clothes and went to the reception to wait. Mother did not say a word.

My husband joined us in time to see the doctor. He explained and interpreted what we already knew and asked us to get admitted to the hospital immediately so that we may have a D&C procedure. We did not know how long I had been living with a dead fetus. It had to be removed urgently. Overstaying with a dead fetus can cause hemorrhage and eventually hemorrhagic shock which leads to death.

We agreed to go home and get ready for the procedure. By evening, we planned to be in the hospital where we would meet our doctor to have the procedure done. Up to this point, there were no tears in my eyes. I had to think about my life be-fore I could process what had just happened. I was not giving up on life, even though life had refused to come out of me.

Besides, I did not know if I could stop my tears if I started shedding them. I was afraid of my own emotions.

When I left the doctor's office, I was very hungry. I kept yawning and asking for food. My mother and I went into an eatery as my husband finished paying the medical bills.

*****

I could see my grief in my mother's eyes. I am sure she was battling her tears too. She knew that her little girl was in pain and saying sorry would not change a thing. She asked me how I felt. I did not answer for quite a while. When I did, I asked her to be stronger than she was. I asked her to put her faith in God since He had not forsaken me. He was very much aware of my pain.

These were the encouraging words that I told people. I believed in them and as I told mother, I hoped she believed in them too. However, my truth at the time was different. I was not strong, I did not have faith and I was sure that I had been forsaken by the one God in whom I had put all my trust. I asked myself questions that I could not voice to anyone.

As we sat down to have our roast potatoes and chicken for lunch, a sudden heat wave engulfed my body. That day I had done some rough cornrow lines on my head and worn an expensive wig on top. My maxi dress was the minimalist's outfit that made me look like a million-dollar girl. The heat quickly spread from the bottom of my body to-wards the top.

"Mum, I do not think I am well," I said to mother.

I was slowly losing control of my body. I could feel my body growing weaker.

"This heat is too much. Take off my clothes mum, pull off my wig. I can't see, mum. I can't … Please hold me. I can't … Help me mum, mum …"Everything went dark in an instant.

My mind told me to let go, to stop fighting and relax my body. I lost consciousness. It felt like I was floating or flying in a dark vacuum space, a truly unexplainable feeling.

The wailing sounds of my mother brought me back to consciousness. I was informed that I had passed out for about five minutes. My mother's wailing was so loud that when I opened my eyes, I gathered some strength amidst my inconsistent breathing pattern, to assure her that I was okay. Other women at the restaurant had left their food and come to my rescue. Some were holding my mother while others administered first aid to me.

I was no longer hungry. Some water and fanning gave me temporary relief as my mother called my doctor, husband, and father.

We went directly to the emergency section of the hospital. In my weak state, I could see the distress on the faces of the nurses when I arrived. They were the same nurses who had attended to me the first time I had a miscarriage. They did not under-stand why I was there again and neither did I. I was admitted and a D & C procedure was done.

The morning after the procedure, the doctor visit-ed with us on our hospital bed. He showed me what had been removed from my womb, which would have been our baby. He explained to me that it was going to the laboratory. Some tests needed to be done to determine what would have caused the unfortunate occurrences.

During our recovery period, it was recommended that we see a therapist and attend counseling sessions. My husband and I did not know what to say to each other. We had kept to ourselves, spending most of our time indoors with each one of us choosing different ways to occupy our minds. For me, I chose movies and television. I needed some-thing interesting to occupy my mind. Any single second that I wasn't distracted, my thoughts gravitated toward my misfortunes resulting in wailing and uncontrolled tears. My husband occupied his mind with work. After we were discharged from the hospital, he stayed in the house for one day then resumed duty when my sister arrived to stay with us. He, however, worked half day and came home early to be with me, only to find himself occupied with newspapers and mobile devices. Any minute away from his device led to deep breaths from him as if he was in deep thoughts which he could not control.

*****

Unlike our first pregnancy, it took us longer to process the reality of what had befallen us. It was impossible to forget, just as it was impossible to forget a deceased friend or relative. The loss is al-ways somewhere in our mind. Not only had we lost a pregnancy, but we had lost two. It was time to take a step back and answer some very difficult questions.

At that time, we remembered a story told to us by our uncle when we visited his house just before we got married. It was a story of the migration of people. In that story, my clansmen seemed to have branched out from my husband's clansmen more than a century or two ago when the Bantu speaking people of Kenya migrated and settled into their current places.

If this story was true, then my husband and I would be relatives and experience some genetic defects that could be causing miscarriages. My clans-men, however, did thorough research on my husband and his people before they allowed us to be married. However, when such things happen, you can't help but wonder.

At the hospital, the results shockingly showed that neither I nor my unborn fetus suffered any abnormality. The doctor advised that we wait for about six months before trying to have another child. He explained to us that we could be experiencing a chromosomal disorder. This too needed to be investigated further.

Six months was never going to be enough for our spirit, let alone our hearts to heal. It would take longer to get to the bottom of the problem we might be experiencing. We also needed to reconcile to the fact that we may never know the cause of our loss. All we needed was to put our faith in God. The same faith that we had before our second miscarriage. Faith seems like a simple act of trust with a small caveat. We trust in a God that we have never seen or met. It is no wonder that it is difficult to love God if you cannot love man. Makes perfect sense since you see man every day but you don't see God. In whatever religion, we rely on God for guidance through our spirit and soul. We put all our hopes and desires in Him.

Our marriage was founded in faith. My husband and I were raised conscious of our Christianity. Our hope was that we would pass that same faith to our children.

Children who we prayed for, planned for and dreamt for. Wouldn't it have been easier to bear children this way?

My husband and I had got into many fights especially on Sundays when he asked me to dress up for church. How could I go to church when God had forsaken me? I asked him why we had to go to church, why he still had the faith and why he did not realize that God had twice abandoned us.

I had spent my entire childhood in church, not just on Sundays but also on other days of the week. I served in the church, I preached the good gospel and even did my humanly best to leave an exemplary life.

At this point, I regretted skipping out on many naughty things that my age mates had done. Things like carefree casual sex on road trips, get-ting too drunk to wake up in the morning and tricking people out of their money. I truly believed that I needed to not only be a perfect example to my siblings but also represent my God well. The same God that I had prayed to when I was carrying my babies. On my second pregnancy, my prayer was very specific, Dear God, my father, father of Abraham, Moses,

Shadrack, Meshack, and Abednego. In your seat, you have seen the pain I have had to bear. Your loving nature has allowed me to carry another, please allow me to hold it in my hands. Please grant me a testimony of your mercies and goodness.

I made this prayer the moment I realized that I was carrying my second pregnancy. Yet here I was, feeling betrayed by my God. How then did my own husband have the guts to ask me to go to church? If God wanted us to know He was there, He would prove Himself as He had all through our lives. Our relationship and faith needed to end, or so I thought.

*****

Many people had asked why we would not just adopt a child. Since my childhood, I knew I would one day adopt a child to raise as my own. That was a fact that was never to be influenced by my ability or inability to bear children. I spent a considerate part of my childhood volunteering in children's homes. I washed, cleaned and helped babysit infants who had been picked in the streets and garbage sites by Good Samaritans. I developed a soft spot for children who had been abandoned and needed help. I had promised myself that should God give me the opportunity, I would adopt one or two such children. I remember having this conversation with my husband just before we got married. It took him a while to accept my vision but he eventually saw the need and accepted it.

This was long before we experienced any miscarriage or lost hope in having our own children. As soon as we began talking about our challenges, people who were oblivious of our future plans started throwing the suggestion to us.

My husband and I did not adopt a child. We did not want to adopt a child just for the mere reason that we could not have our own.

Adopting a child just because we could not have a child of our own sounded selfish. What if we took this child and then got our own? Would we love it the same way? The intentions and motivation had to be right.

For us, any person adopting a child should have clear and selfless intentions. Those intentions should be nothing but to give the child a permanent home, love and sufficient provision.

Looking back, the pain of losing a child made me understand how a motherless child feels. During my grieving period, I felt an emptiness that is be-yond explanation. I felt alone and betrayed. I imagined that was what children felt when abandoned in a bin instead of being in their mother's hands. They must feel an emptiness greater than mine, for I have known a mother's love, I thought. For this rea-son, we felt it was safe that motherless children were adopted by people who understood the rea-sons for adopting children. They should be adopted to homes complete with parents; homes where they were wanted and loved unconditionally.

*****

As a young girl, I saw my great grandmother give her service to the church. Even in her old age, church elders would often visit to check on her and pray with her. She was committed to Christ. Her love and commitment to people were also evident for all to see.

How had she survived past the shame and abandonment? How could she commit to a God that had clearly shamed her in a society where a woman was defined by the number of children she bore? It must have been worse for her than it was for me.

After recovery, my husband and I were open to talking about our difficulties. I was stigmatized and singled out for my struggles. Once, a friend suggested that I had been cursed. Another insensitively asked if I had procured any abortions before I was married. Others simply stopped inviting us to their children's celebrations. They felt we would bring a somber mood to their celebrations.

I was conscious of the whispers around me. One of my friends once expressed her disappointment in my decision to wait until after my wedding so as to have children. "What's the point of waiting until marriage only to learn that you have complications?" she asked bluntly, "You should have be-come pregnant before marriage"

Many friends and relatives became a threat to our marriage. My husband received a lot of advice, some urged him to out rightly leave me for another woman.

"There are many women in this world, why stick with the one who can't give you an heir? You are not getting any younger," they advised.

"She must be feeding you the wrong types of food. You are an African man, you must eat right in order to sire," others chipped in ignorantly.

We had to shut our ears and trust our love and friendship to pull us through the tough times.

We guarded ourselves because we knew what we meant to each other and why we got married. Our priority was to ourselves and not to the intrusive society around us.

We have since learned to live past all the comments thrown at us. I read a certain quote which said; if you cannot change it why stress about it? If I could not place a child in my womb and cause it to stay there for nine months, why should I stress about it?

I chose to speak about my struggles so that other women could come out and share their struggles and fight the stigma from society. While we could not control what others thought of us, what we thought of ourselves was entirely up to us.

The fact that I was with a man who cared for me more than for his need to have children was com-forting enough. Severally I had asked myself how easy it would have been for him to leave his matrimonial home and have a child with another woman. Besides, I do not look as beautiful as I did when we met. Then I had a perfect Body to Mass Index (BMI). I could easily balance in a six-inch stiletto. My hairline was intact and my eyes hopeful and brighter.

I am bigger in size now and no longer wear my stilettos comfortably. My stunningly good looks have since been replaced by wisdom and wit. I dream different, I reason differently. The woman my husband knew years ago is long gone. Every day he meets a new woman in me, a woman with similar roots with the one he met yesterday, but who keeps evolving and growing by the day.

For him, I came first. He did his best to be there for me and to love me even when I was difficult. We had enough in each other and I couldn't be more grateful.

*****

It is one thing for someone to believe in you and another to believe in yourself. It is also easier to disappoint another person than yourself because our human nature has us selfishly thinking about ourselves. Apart from becoming a mother and a wife, I had so many dreams as a young girl. I wanted to be a career woman, a successful one at that. I wanted to be a true friend and confidant.

Life is however like one long stretch of road. One day you are moving smoothly and the next you are so roughly shaken that you lose focus of where you are headed. Sometimes you stop to catch a breath and forget to keep moving. My difficulties in bearing children were not only sapping away my energy but also making me forget how wholesome life is meant to be. It was taking me too long to over-come my challenges, too long to continue with my journey of becoming. I was willing to shut my eyes and keep still through the rest of the journey of life.

The stillness, however, made me realize that every-thing that had previously happened in my life had played a great role in the person I had become; Boarding school had shaped my character, my relationship with my parents had shaped my persona and the exposure I received had made me a bold and fearless woman.

I was beginning to see that something good might actually come out of my struggles. Maybe I was being prepared for parenthood and the value that comes with having a child in a fast-paced society. Who knows what lessons today's struggles have for tomorrow?

As I waited, I made up my mind to become the best version of myself. To chase after my dreams and become that which I intentionally wanted to be. I decided that the journey of life would continue in the best way I possibly could direct it.

*****

We opened our home to visitors when we got over our struggles. My husband and I are both people oriented. We, therefore, loved to host our friends and family in our home. One day, my brother called and asked to see us. He wanted to officially bring her fiancée to our home. Even though we knew her, she had never visited. My brother wanted her to feel part of the family as they planned their union. We were happy to have them.

The morning before they arrived, I went to the market and bought my brother's favorite meal.

We had such a wonderful time catching up. They came bearing good news, they were having a baby. This good news caught me by surprise. At first, I thought it was a prank, but when they insisted it wasn't, I was elated.

Somehow my heart was filled and my hope renewed. This news pushed me to believe in God again because as much as I had lost my faith, I felt that He was speaking to me directly through my brother. His message was clear. I was just not listening. He had not forgotten about me.

That day I learned a lesson that no teacher or personal experience would ever teach; to accept the things that are beyond me. I learned to let go and live my best life. I learned not to focus on the pain or let a dark cloud hover over my head and steal my joy. I felt that my husband, my family, and the world deserved the best version of me today, after all, tomorrow is never promised.

I made it a priority to pray for the safe delivery of my niece. My sister and I bought all the toys and children's clothes that we found along our way. We knew we were going to spoil her, make her the epitome of our lives. Our first family baby arrived safely and brought so much joy to the family. She was named after our mother. We hoped and prayed that she would take all the good traits that our mother possessed.

*****

Names have power. What you name your child is said to have weight on what that child becomes. Some communities name their children after sea-sons, others after long gone relatives. Some com-munities leave room for creativity and come up with new names, and others, in special cases like myself, name their children after important people in their lives.

I sometimes wonder what was going through my great grandmother's mind when she asked that I be named after her. Did she know what I would become or the burdens I would have to bear? When she first held me in her arms and made ululations of joy to celebrate my birth, had she blessed me as old women did? Did she unknowingly also bless me with a curse? Gaudenzia had six children, two of them males and four females.

When she died, they were all grownups with their own lineage. On the day of her burial, there was a requiem ser-vice held in her honor at the local church. A send-off ceremony was then done under a huge mango tree in her compound, now the compound of my grandfather's younger brother. The tree, to date, is still very fruitful, it has low hanging branches with seasonal fresh and juicy mangoes. Anyone who has had the privilege of walking or sitting under the shade of this tree has enjoyed the goodness of its mangoes.

During her burial, old women and men cried for her. They called her by name and wailed asking why she had to leave. They spoke to her corpse as if she was there. Boiled and salted maize and beans were eaten to celebrate her life, roasted nuts and black tea was also in plenty. She was laid to rest in her grave that was next to her husband's grave, in front of their hut.

On that day, I was least bothered. I did not cry nor say goodbye. I was too young to understand the weight of what was happening. I continued playing with my age mates, unmoved. I was clumsy, I did not keep still, just as I had not kept still years before when she wanted me to sit next to her under a similar mango tree in my grandfather's compound. That day I did not realize I had lost the one woman who would have told me all I needed to know about myself. Now, I am like a budding tree, sprouting through the pain and fighting all odds to become.

#THE END